I0409249

Don't Diet, Live It!

A yearlong inspiration for a healthy life that is attainable, sustainable, and fun!

Dyan Damron

Cover photo & design by Jacob Cleaver

A healthy life does not involve restrictions or overindulgence. We just have to find our happy healthy place with all things in moderation. Obesity is not caused by eating one piece of cake or by skipping one day of exercise. Obesity is caused by allowing those daily choices to become our lifestyle.

By opening this book, you are already on your way to living your healthy happy life! I am so proud of you for realizing you can stop dieting and start living. Turn the page and keep up the good work!

Introduction

This book is a summary of my research, trials, choices, mistakes, and triumphs. I found what works and what doesn't because I lived through it. I know that a healthy life can be attainable, sustainable, and fun. I stopped dieting and started living. And this book will prove that you can too!

Each chapter represents a month of the year. You can start this book, just like you can choose to change your life, at any moment, on any day, in any year. My stories, recipes, and fitness tips are meant to inspire you. They are not rules – they are motivators. They are not trendy – they are timeless.

I encourage you to try my recipes and meal ideas as inspiration. If you are missing an ingredient, leave it out. If your family prefers raspberries over strawberries, broccoli over asparagus, or chicken over fish, swap it out. And I also urge you to get the entire family – kids and adults – involved. You are never too young or too old to cook in the kitchen or get physically active!

I am a woman who has been overweight. I was teased as a child for being chubby and starved myself only to end up binge eating. I struggled with cellulite and stretch marks and fought my own demons. Through it all I finally learned how to get healthy, feel good, and be satisfied with myself. I lost 50 pounds and have kept it off for over a decade. During that decade I survived numerous personal losses, tragedies, and heartaches. The one thing I know, had I not lost the weight and learned how to love and respect myself, I would have never survived.

I now feel my mission is to help others regain their lives. This calling is why I left my corporate job in 2010 and started Coach D Consulting. I have helped friends, coworkers, family, and clients lose weight, eliminate medications, sleep better, look great, and feel amazing. I have proven to be successful and now I want to help as many people as I can. It is my passion to help others live a healthy happy life.

Obesity is so frustrating because it is a 100% preventable epidemic that is killing us at an alarming rate. But you can use this book as a step in the right direction. You can pick up this book any day of the year and find inspiration, words of encouragement, and ideas for fitness and food. I ask you to join me each day and make a change for the better. By the end of the year you will have added years to your life and life to your years!

Chapter 1: January

New Year, New Day, New Chance

Each New Year, many of us make resolutions. We make a pledge to ourselves that we will reinvent or transform into a better, faster, stronger, less cursing, more praising, highly philanthropic, in-the-moment person. While our intentions may be good, our goals are often too lofty and our willpower is too low. It's been said "the road to hell is paved with good intentions", and without a good plan, determination, and support, many of us will fail or abandon our resolutions. In fact, only about 50% of people keep their New Year's resolutions for three months, and even less keep them for six months.

Some of the top resolutions each year include losing weight, getting in shape, and eating healthier. These are awesome long-term goals. However, we must first make a plan and achieve short-term goals so that we can realize our long-term resolutions. So many times we don't stick to our resolutions, especially when it comes to weight loss or health because we put unrealistic limitations and expectations on ourselves. Don't resolve to go on a diet or try a fitness gimmick, resolve to change your life and be healthy. Here are my tips to help you fulfill your resolution for a healthy year.

<u>*Be Realistic*</u>: If you haven't run farther than across a parking lot in the past year, chances are you won't be running a half-marathon this spring. And if you haven't been to a gym since...you're not even sure when, chances are you aren't going to become a gym rat anytime soon. Make weekly goals that you can accomplish – take a 20-minute walk around the block after dinner, add one vegetable to each meal, go to bed 10 minutes earlier and get up 10 minutes earlier to do jumping jacks and pushups. Once you've met that goal, set an additional one for the next week.

Make a schedule: We put meetings, practices, lunches, etc in our calendar. Make yourself a priority and write (or type) your workouts, grocery trips, and food prep days into your calendar. You wouldn't cancel a meeting with your boss or miss your kid's game, so don't be a no-show to yourself!

Stay Positive: Chances are you will have a bad day and you will make a bad choice. But, don't let it get you down. Remember your long-term goals and realize that one little hiccup does not mean you should throw in the towel. Tomorrow (or the next meal) is a new chance to make a better decision. No matter what, you can always get back on track. Each new day is a new chance for a fresh start.

Ask for Help: We are more likely to stick to our resolutions when we have a partner to hold us accountable. So pick someone you trust and share your resolution, goals, and plan. Be specific about what you need, and ask them to motivate you and help you stay on track. Choose someone that will hold you responsible, but will not criticize or make you feel worse.

Celebrate Your Success: When you've accomplished one of your short-term goals, it is important to reward yourself. But be careful that the reward doesn't undo what you've accomplished. Rather than celebrating with food, do something that makes you feel good and boosts confidence. Get a mani/pedi or massage, buy a new pair of running shoes or workout gear, take a new class, or get a new kitchen gadget (a new blender for smoothies or indoor grill pan for fish and veggies).

   With these tips I know you will be successful in the coming year. This can be your healthiest year yet. And don't think January 1st is the only day you can make a change. Each new day is a new opportunity – a fresh start and chance to get healthy. Make today the day you decide to live better, look better, and feel better. Obesity is 100% preventable and this is the New Year, new day, and new chance to make it happen!

It Takes Two to Make a Thing Go Right

If you're making a New Year's resolution, make it a two-pronged approach. Remember the 80's funk song from Rob Base & DJ EZ Rock? They had it right – it does take two. Both nutrition and exercise are needed to keep you healthy. Good nutrition and exercise together are shown to reduce the size of abdominal fat cells (the most dangerous ones around your middle which are linked to higher triglycerides and increased risk for heart disease). Only doing one will not reduce those abdominal fat cells. Plus, exercising has a ripple effect on your entire body – your muscles become more efficient at using blood, your heart gets stronger, and your blood vessels become more limber so blood flows more easily. This means that you not only look better, but more importantly, you feel better.

You don't have to run a marathon to get these benefits. Cardiologists recommend getting an average of 30 minutes of aerobic activity every day. This amount of exercise can increase your life expectancy by 3½ years! In addition, a study out of the Cooper Institute in Dallas found that even moderately fit people had half the death rates of those who were sedentary. Your 30 minutes of activity don't necessarily have to come at one time during the day. Take three 10-minute walks throughout the day. Or, wake up 15 minutes early for a quick walk before you hit the shower – I guarantee you will feel better all day. Then, take a walk around the block with a family member (or the dog) after dinner.

We all want to be healthy so we can live long and prosperous lives. If it means you have more years to spend with your family, who wouldn't be willing to eat healthy and exercise? So tell yourself and your family, "It takes two to make a thing go right. It takes two to make it outta sight. Hit it!"

My Don't Diet, Live It Meal for this month is a nice departure from the heavy holiday fare we've all had over the past few months. Shake things up with a fresh Mexican fiesta! Many Mexican meals consist of fried tortillas, fatty cheese sauces, and refried beans made with lard. But, Mexican food doesn't have to weigh you down. This meal is a fresh take on all our favorites, minus the added fat and calories. If you're making this on New Year's Day and want a little Southern tradition, substitute black-eyed peas for the black beans! This meal is perfect for the entire family and much of it can be done ahead – even the day before! The following recipes serve four.

Fiesta Fish Tacos

Ingredients:
1 lb firm white fish filets (cod, halibut, mahi, tilapia, or haddock)
Seasoning for fish: ½ t cumin, ½ t chili powder, ½ t salt, ¼ t pepper, ¼ t smoked paprika, pinch of cayenne pepper
1 T extra virgin olive oil (EVOO)
1 head of red cabbage, shredded (or bag of coleslaw mix)
¼ cup red onion, thinly sliced
Juice of 2 limes
2 t agave syrup
1 T vinegar (red or white wine)
½ t salt, ¼ t pepper
8-12 whole grain or corn tortillas (small size 4-6-inch diameter)
1 avocado, 1 cup lowfat sour cream, 2 T finely chopped cilantro
Directions:
Prepare cabbage ahead (at least a few hours or day before) by combining cabbage, red onion, juice of 1 lime, agave, vinegar, salt, and pepper. Allow to sit in fridge until ready to serve.
Prepare fish ahead (at least 30 minutes or day before) by cutting filets into ½-inch x 3-inch strips and pat dry with paper towel. Dust with seasoning and allow to rest in fridge. Preheat oven to 400 degrees. Line a baking sheet with foil and spread with EVOO. Place fish strips on pan and bake for 5-8 minutes, or until fish is firm and browned slightly around edges.

While fish is cooking, wrap tortillas in foil and put in oven for last minute of cooking to warm and make more pliable.

Serve fish immediately on platter. Make a "taco bar" with fish, tortillas, cabbage, avocado, sour cream, and cilantro. Everyone can choose what and how much they want of each item. It's fun, flavorful, and super healthy. Plus, fish provides benefits to our hearts, minds, and bodies. Who knew a fiesta could be so healthy!

Black Bean and Corn Salsa

Ingredients:
1 T EVOO
1 cup frozen corn, thawed and drained
1 can black beans, rinsed and drained
4 plum tomatoes, seeded and diced
¼ cup red onion, finely diced
1 jalapeño, ribs and seeds removed, finely diced
½ t salt, ¼ t pepper
Directions:
Heat EVOO in a large skillet on med-high heat, add corn and allow to brown slightly. Remove from heat and allow to cool. Add remaining ingredients. You can serve at room temp, or make ahead (up to a couple days) and serve cold. It can be used as a salsa with tacos, or even as a side dish or salad. It's delicious and loaded with fiber and antioxidants!

Strawberrita

Ingredients:
2 cups frozen strawberries, thawed
1 T agave syrup
Juice of 4 limes, plus zest of 1 lime
1 cup water (for nonalcoholic) OR 1 cup silver tequila or rum
1 cup ice
4 fresh strawberries, optional

Directions:
Combine ingredients in a blender until smooth (leave out ice for "on the rocks"). Pour into a fun glass and serve with a fresh strawberry for garnish. A cocktail with a bonus – one cup of strawberries contains over 100 mg of vitamin C, almost as much as a cup of orange juice! Who needs OJ when you can have a 'rita!

Un-fried Ice Cream

Ingredients:
4 scoops vanilla frozen yogurt
1 cup low-sugar cereal (Bran Flakes, Cheerios, Crispix, Wheat Chex, or Shredded Wheat)
2 t cinnamon
1 cup frozen strawberries, thawed
1 T agave syrup
Directions:
Prepare frozen yogurt ahead (at least 2 hours, up to 2 days before) by scooping 4 scoops onto a small pan or plate. Place back in freezer. Add cereal and cinnamon to a baggie. Crush with a pan or meat mallet. Pour into a bowl. Roll frozen scoops in crumbs until evenly coated and refreeze until ready to serve (cover with plastic if more than 2 hours).
Prepare syrup ahead (up to 2 days) by adding berries and agave to blender. Puree until smooth – add a bit of water if needed to thin.
Serve cereal-covered scoops in a cocktail glass or fun bowl and drizzle with strawberry syrup. It's crunchy (but not deep-fried), and it's loaded with calcium and vitamins!

Chapter 2: February

The Love of Your Life

When Valentine's Day rolls around, most of us are thinking of ways we can show our significant other how much we love him or her. However, I suggest we all take the time to also show ourselves a little love. While I have been known to be a bit of a cynic when it comes to finding romance with "the one", I am certainly no skeptic when it comes to being true to the only person you'll be with forever – yourself. And honestly, how can you expect someone else to love you if you don't love yourself. Plus, if you don't take care of yourself, you won't be around for all those future Valentine's Days to show and receive love from another.

In this nipped, tucked, and Botoxed world of reality television and air-brushed advertisements, many people get a warped sense of beauty and what they think they should look like. However, this Valentine's Day, I encourage women and men of all ages to look in the mirror and embrace what you see. You shouldn't starve yourself to fit into some skimpy dress or skinny jeans. And no one should want to erase the minor flaws that come from living a full life. Look in the mirror and truly love what you see. The wrinkles and crow's feet around your eyes echo the laughter you have shared over the years. The wrinkles around your lips are mementos of the kisses you have given to show affection. The stretch marks are a token of the way your body beautifully adapted to bear your child. And those few extra pounds you've added over the decades are evidence of the many birthday cakes, holiday meals, and boxes of chocolates you have shared with the ones you love. The freckles and dark spots on your skin are a reflection of the hours of fun you spent playing in the sun.

Why would anyone want to take away all those beautiful memories? Chances are, your significant other loves your true beauty and recognizes that they are memories and not flaws. And remember to tell your significant other this Valentine's Day how beautiful they are and how much you love them. And whether you have a significant other or not, remember that YOU are the love of your life – your own life. Look in the mirror and love yourself. Know that you need to take care of your body and stay healthy – no one else can do that for you.

So this year celebrate Valentine's Day and enjoy that box of chocolates – just maybe stick to the small box and make it dark chocolate this year! Obesity is 100% preventable and it starts with the love of your life!

Move for Your Body and Your Beauty

Just a 30-minute walk each day can do wonders for your health. But it can also boost your beauty! Here's how:

- *For your complexion: Like all cardiovascular exercise, walking gets your heart pumping and improves circulation. And better blood flow means your skin (the largest organ of the body) receives plenty of the nutrient-rich blood it needs for optimal health. Wrinkles and age spots aren't attractive! The sun is always beating down on us, even in these colder winter months. Help prevent wrinkles by walking!*

- *For your bones: Weight-bearing exercise such as walking and jogging helps build bone mass, which can fend off osteoporosis. Brittle bones and poor posture are not sexy!*

Hopefully you get plenty of exercise for internal health – to feel better and live longer, but even a little vanity should give you incentive to get your workout on!

My Don't Diet, Live It Meal for February is good for the heart! After all, February is American Heart Month. So while you decorate cards with hearts, keep your heart healthy by preparing a meal for yourself and all those you "heart". I have chosen an Italian meal for this month since Mediterranean cuisine is most well-known for being heart-healthy. So, take a romantic trip to Italy without leaving your kitchen! The following recipes serve four.

Salmon Puttanesca with Lentils

Ingredients:
2 cups water
1 cup lentils, rinsed
4 (6 ounces each) salmon fillets, skin and bones removed
½ t salt, ¼ t pepper
2 T extra virgin olive oil (EVOO)
½ cup diced onion
2 T capers
¼ cup rough-chopped pitted kalamata or black olives
2 T chopped garlic
2 t tomato paste
¼ t red pepper flakes (optional if feeding kids)
1 (14.5-ounce) can no-salt-added diced tomatoes
2 T red wine vinegar
Juice of 1 lemon
1 T chopped basil

Directions:
Preheat the oven to 325 degrees. Add water and lentils to a small saucepan. Bring to a boil, then reduce the heat to a simmer and cook for 15 minutes. Drain and set aside.
Season the salmon fillets with salt and pepper. In a large nonstick sauté pan, heat 1 T of EVOO over med-high heat and add the salmon fillets. Cook for 3 minutes, then turn and cook for 1-2 minutes on the other side. Remove the fillets to a baking sheet fitted with a rack and put in the oven.

Add the remaining 1 T of EVOO to the same pan, over high heat. Add the onions, capers, and olives. Stir until the onions just starting to caramelize. Add the garlic, tomato paste, and red pepper flakes and sauté for 2 minutes more. Stir in the tomatoes, red wine vinegar and lemon juice. Reduce the heat to a simmer and cook for 3-4 minutes. Add the lentils and stir in basil and remove from heat.

Remove the salmon from oven. Serve salmon atop the lentil and Puttanesca sauce. Garnish with basil leaves, if desired.

Unfamiliar with lentils? They are dried beans that are relatively quick and easy to prepare. A small but mighty member of the legume family, lentils are a very good source of cholesterol-lowering fiber, and also provide six important minerals, two B-vitamins, and protein – all with virtually no fat. Plus, salmon is an excellent source of omega-3 – a fabulous fat that improves brain function and improves hair, skin, and nails! A yummy and nutritional powerhouse of a meal!

Sparkling Lemonade

Ingredients:
32 ounces sparkling or seltzer water
Juice of 4 lemons
4 t agave syrup
Lemon slices for garnish (optional)
Ice
Directions:
In individual glass or large pitcher, squeeze juice of lemons and muddle (crush with end of wooden spoon) with agave and ice. Pour chilled sparkling water over mixture. Add a lemon slice on top or hang over rim of glass. Tangy and delicious! For adult enjoyment, add a shot of vodka or substitute champagne instead of sparkling water.

Lemons contain unique flavonoid compounds that have antioxidant and anti-cancer properties. It's tangy, refreshing, and good for you!

Affogato Sundae

Ingredients:
2 cups vanilla frozen yogurt
4 T brewed coffee or espresso (substitute vanilla extract for young kids)
4 T amaretto liqueur (omit for kids)
4 graham crackers or gingersnap cookies
¼ cup sliced almonds
Directions:
Place a ½ cup scoop of frozen yogurt into a bowl. Top each with 1 T coffee and liqueur (or dash of vanilla). Stick a graham cracker or gingersnap on side of each scoop and sprinkle with almonds.

Coffee is loaded with antioxidants. Almonds help lower cholesterol and are super heart healthy. Plus, yogurt offers calcium and vitamins as well as live bacterial cultures that help you to live longer, and may fortify your immune system. Dessert anyone?

Chapter 3: March

Spring Ahead, Propel Forward

The arrival of March means that Memorial Day weekend is only about 12 weeks away. That means that the official start to summer will be here before we know it. March also means that we will set our clocks one hour ahead in anticipation of longer days, warmer mornings, and hotter nights. As we set our clocks ahead, let this also be the time that we propel ourselves forward. In the short time we have between now and Memorial Day weekend, we will have some pretty major events – spring break, spring weddings, Easter, prom, and a host of other warm weather activities.

Winter can be especially brutal. Between the cold weather and the threat of flu, most of us have been hibernating and wrapped up in layers. Chances are underneath those layers, we may be hiding some extra weight that is not quite ready for wedding or prom dresses, and certainly not bathing suits. But have no fear, with a little hard work and determination, you can be ready to shed the layers and look fantastic in whatever attire spring and summer brings your way.

I know personally how scary the thought of spring break, bathing suits, pools, and beaches can be. I can remember hating the idea of trying on bathing suits each spring. Trying to find the one that would hide my belly rolls or cover my hips was an annual routine. And I can remember trying to find just the right cover up so I wouldn't feel terribly embarrassed standing next to my thin high school friends at the pool. I would practice how to cross my arms or position my legs so that I could hide excess weight or cover cellulite. I tried diets, but they just didn't work. I would starve myself for a couple days only to end up eating cookie dough straight from the container.

I was in college when I finally learned how to eat well, exercise properly, and respect my body. I eventually lost 50 pounds by completely changing my lifestyle. It didn't happen overnight, but I saw measurable results each week. And I can remember one day looking in the mirror and finally seeing a body that I loved, respected, and felt secure about. My body image was no longer one of self-doubt, ridicule, and agony. I transformed my body image to be one of strength, beauty, and confidence. I wish I had known more at an earlier age about healthy living. It would have saved me a lot of heartache.

My struggle made me stronger. And I now give you my knowledge and strength so you can achieve success. Obesity is 100% preventable and this spring is your time to propel forward!

Put a Spring in Your Step

With the warmer temps outside, it will soon be time to hit the pool...and yes, that means a bathing suit! So, it's time to break a sweat now! But think cardio is the best way to lose weight? Consider this: resistance training, or weight lifting, can actually be more effective at fighting the flab. Studies have shown that 72 hours after lifting weights, your resting calorie burn will be increased by 7.9%. And a study published in Medicine & Science in Sports & Exercise *showed that women who lifted a challenging weight for eight reps burned nearly twice as many calories as women who knocked out 15 reps with lighter dumbbells. Many women avoid resistance training for fear of bulking up, but it just won't happen – natural female hormones prevent muscle development like a man.*

Plus, a pound of fat burns about 2 calories per day, while a pound of muscle burns about 6 calories per day. Another bonus: one pound of fat takes up 18% more space on your body than one pound of muscle. So, lift weights to drop the pounds and look more slender! It is a great way to increase metabolism and show off some muscle definition – just in time for the pool!

My Don't Diet, Live It Meal for March utilizes all the freshness and ripeness of the spring season. When you use seasonal ingredients, they will taste the best and will be most affordable. These scrumptious springtime supper recipes serve four – great for entertaining or dinner with the family! Buy in-season and use double-duty ingredients to save money!

Asparagus, Salmon and Goat Cheese Frittata

Ingredients:
2 t extra virgin olive oil (EVOO)
1 T chopped garlic
¼ cup finely diced shallot or onion
8 asparagus spears
¼ cup crumbled goat cheese
2 ounces smoked salmon (or Nova lox)
½ t salt, ¼ t pepper
6 large eggs
¼ cup lowfat sour cream
½ t cayenne pepper
1 T hot sauce (or 1 t red wine vinegar)
2 T water

Directions:
Preheat oven to 340 degrees. Prepare 1½ quart Pyrex dish (or glass pie pan or muffin tin) with non-stick cooking spray.

Sauté first three ingredients in a non-stick skillet over medium heat until onions are translucent. Add asparagus and sauté for an additional 2-3 minutes (less time needed if stalks are thin). Remove from heat and add to baking dish – evenly spread along bottom. Crumble goat cheese and salmon over asparagus mixture and sprinkle with salt and pepper.

Add eggs, sour cream, cayenne, hot sauce, and water to a blender and mix on high for one minute (the mixture will nearly double in volume). Gently pour egg mixture over asparagus, cheese, and salmon. Bake for 30-40 minutes, depending on how soft you prefer your eggs. Allow to rest before slicing.

Use this base recipe as a method – you can use any veggies and meat combination you like. Some of my favorites are ham, Swiss, and arugula; tomato, mozzarella, and spinach; turkey or chicken sausage, roasted red bell peppers, and Monterey jack.

This recipe is great for breakfast, lunch, dinner, or even a high-protein snack. It tastes great hot, warm, room temp, or even straight from the fridge! Refrigerate leftovers for up to a week. It's cheerful, cheap, and loaded with protein and antioxidants!

Berry Almond Salad

<u>Ingredients</u>:
4 T EVOO
2 T red wine vinegar
½ t salt, ¼ t pepper
6 cups baby greens – spinach, arugula, or spring mix
¼ cup goat cheese
½ cup sliced almonds
½ cup fresh raspberries, blueberries, or combination
<u>Directions</u>:
Whisk (or use food processor to get extra creamy) first three ingredients together to make dressing. In a large serving bowl, top greens with dressing and toss. Add remaining ingredients and toss again. Serve alongside frittata. It's full of texture and a wholesome salad that everyone will love!

Iced Fruit Tea

<u>Ingredients</u>:
1 quart fresh brewed black or green tea – chilled
2 lemons
½ cup fresh raspberries, plus a few for garnish
Ice
<u>Directions</u>:
In individual glass or large pitcher, muddle (crush with end of wooden spoon) juice of one lemon, raspberries, and ice. Pour chilled tea over fruit and ice and serve with lemon wedge and a few fresh raspberries. Sweet! And you don't need to add sugar!

Souped-Up Sorbet

<u>Ingredients</u>:
Raspberry sorbet or sherbet
4 dark chocolate squares or 4 T dark chocolate chips (at least 70% cacao)
Fresh raspberries for garnish
<u>Directions</u>:
Add one scoop of sorbet to a martini glass (or other decorative dish). Stick one dark chocolate square into the sorbet (or use vegetable peeler to shave chocolate on top) or sprinkle 1 T chocolate chips and add a few fresh raspberries to garnish! Very gourmet, but super easy...and healthful!

Chapter 4: April

Spring In To the Season

I love springtime. It is a season of change and new beginnings. We start heading outdoors, getting more active, eating fresher foods, and truly feeling a new season upon us. I think it is a perfect time for change in our lives as well. I thoroughly enjoy helping parents and their children make lifestyle changes to get them healthier and happier. And what better place to start than with the first holiday of the spring season – Easter!

The celebration of Easter began as a religious holiday in ancient times. It is a "festival" in the Christian calendar that marks the end of Lent and Holy Week. However, nowhere in history did any of the ancient Christians, Greeks, or Jews require that Easter be celebrated with an Easter basket filled to the brim with sugar-loaded candy and fat-packed chocolate! The idea that holidays must include unhealthy foods can lead kids to feel that sugary fatty foods are a celebration and a reward. This is not a behavior we want our kids to grow up with. So, this Easter season, celebrate with fun and healthful treats. I love the idea of an Easter basket, just cram it full of wholesome treats and activities. Here are a few of my suggestions for tossing into your kids' Easter baskets:

- Fill up with apples, oranges, and bananas.
- Costume jewelry, bubbles, stuffed animals, reading or coloring books, box cars make entertaining basket items.
- Toiletries, beauty and grooming products, and scented lotions are fun ways kids can feel pampered without being spoiled.
- To get them in the kitchen, give them their very own whisk, spatula, or vegetable peeler, and maybe even a key ingredient they will need to make their very own lunch or dinner. When kids have ownership they are more likely to eat a healthful meal or snack. Plus, when you make the food yourself, you control the quality of ingredients that your kids eat.

- Homemade gift certificates or coupons for family time. You choose whatever activities your family likes – e.g. one hour of playing their favorite outdoor game, going bowling or playing Wii on rainy days, setting up a tent in the backyard for a "camping" trip, etc.

All things should be enjoyed in moderation, so always toss in a few of their favorite candies on the top of the basket. But, keep them small (no giant bunnies) and individually portioned. A few good options are Peeps, Tootsie Rolls, Cadbury Crème Eggs, and Jelly Beans.

Just Breathe

As many of us know, springtime brings beautiful blooms and plenty of allergies. But you can fight them. Regular exercise can control allergies by creating a strong blood flow. This moves the allergens through the body to the kidneys and the skin, where they are eliminated. A sluggish blood flow tends to allow allergens to settle so they become sedentary and begin to destroy the tissues around them. By continually moving the allergens through the blood they have far less time to inflame the tissues. Regular exercise expels allergens from the body.

In addition to physically breathing better, exercise can help you mentally breathe easier. Exercise leads to changes in the brain that strengthen your resolve against stress because it boosts your brain's production of endorphins – those "feel-good" chemicals. A 20-minute sweat session can be enough to perk up your mood for a whopping 12 hours, reports a University of Vermont study. It may also be as effective as medication for treating depression in some people. In fact, clinically depressed people reported feeling less tense, tired, angry, and confused after a mere 10-minute walk, according to a Duke University study. So do a little heavy breathing to breathe easy!

Most of all, enjoy the holiday with your family. Remember that Easter is a festival, but it doesn't have to be a fat-loaded feast to have fun! Obesity is 100% preventable and it starts by springing in to the season!

My Don't Diet, Live It Meal for Easter is my take on a traditional Easter and springtime meal. I have simplified some Greek fare to make it accessible, healthful, and family-friendly. Lamb is traditional for Easter and spring, but if the bold flavor or cost of lamb is too much for you, scallops are a great alternative and pair nicely with all the flavors in each dish. Once again, use in-season and double-duty ingredients to save money and time, and to keep the theme. The following recipes serve four.

Mixed-Grill Kabobs with Greek-style Dip and Pitas

Ingredients:
1 lb lamb loin or leg OR 1 lb scallops
Choose 2 or 3 different colored veggies from the following:
1 container cherry tomatoes, 2 bell peppers, 1 red onion, 2 zucchini, 2 squash, 1 container button mushrooms, 8 small red-skin potatoes
2 T extra virgin olive oil (EVOO)
1 t salt, ½ t pepper
Skewers (if using wood, soak in water for 1 hr prior to cooking)
4 whole grain pitas
1 cup lowfat plain Greek yogurt or lowfat sour cream
Juice of 1 lime
1 t garlic powder
1 T finely chopped fresh mint (optional)
Directions:
Prepare Greek-style dip by whisking together last five ingredients. You can make this dip the night before or morning of and leave in fridge to allow flavors to develop.
If using lamb, cut into 1-inch cubes. Dry lamb or scallops with a paper towel and set on plate. Drizzle with 1 T EVOO and season with ½ t salt and ¼ t pepper. Skewer meat and set aside.

Rinse and dry veggies and cut into 1-inch cubes (all veggies should be about the same size to ensure even cooking – tomatoes can be left whole). Set on plate and drizzle with 1 T EVOO and season with ½ t salt and ¼ t pepper. Skewer veggies. Keep meat and veggies separate because they will not cook for the same amount of time and this will prevent cross-contamination. You can prepare skewers in advance and leave in fridge for several hours. Grill (indoors or out) or broil skewers for few minutes on each side, rotating once – do not overcook lamb or scallops or they will be tough. Place pitas on grill or under broiler for 30 seconds to warm through. Serve skewers with dip and pitas. Pitas can be used as utensils or you can stuff them with meat, veggies, and dip! Just have fun and enjoy the healthful flavors of the season.

Fizzy Limeades

<u>Ingredients</u>:
32 ounces soda water
2-4 limes
4 t agave syrup
Fresh mint sprigs (optional)
Ice
<u>Directions</u>:
In individual glass or large pitcher, squeeze juice of lime and then muddle (crush with end of wooden spoon) lime, agave, mint, and ice. Pour chilled soda water over mixture. Tangy and delicious! For adult enjoyment, add a shot of vodka or silver tequila! Now that's refreshment!

Pineapple Kabobs

<u>Ingredients</u>:
1 pineapple (peeled and cored whole pineapple in the produce section is same price as fresh)
Skewers (soak wood)
1 cup lowfat vanilla Greek yogurt
4 graham crackers or gingersnap cookies
<u>Directions</u>:
Cut pineapple into 2-inch cubes and skewer. Grill or broil on high heat for about 1-2 minutes on each side. You want to caramelize, but not cook pineapple. Serve with a small scoop of yogurt and sprinkle with crushed graham cracker or gingersnap. Yummy! Added benefit is pineapple contains bromelain, which aids in digesting protein.
Yogurt contains probiotics or "good" bacteria that aid in digestion and immune function. Always pick Greek yogurt, which contains twice the protein and half the sugar as conventional yogurt. And stick with lowfat or fat free versions that say "live and active cultures" on the label. Yogurt also provides a dose of calcium, vitamins B-2 and B-12, potassium, and magnesium.

Chapter 5: May

Mother's Day Reminds Us to Nourish and Care

With Mother's Day this month, I think about all the things we do as a result of our mother's influence. We were all brought into this world by a mother and most of us were raised by a mother. On Mother's Day, some of us celebrate and thank our mothers for their role in raising us. Some of us will be celebrated for giving birth to, or raising, children. And what a lovely day to have on the calendar – a holiday to celebrate the women who have influenced our lives.

I have worked with lots of mothers. As a mom, she will typically say that her final impetus to ask for my help was when she realized she wanted to be a better influence for her kids so they would grow up to be healthy. A mother wants her kids' eating habits as teens and adults to reflect the good choices she taught them while they are still young. Entire families can enjoy healthy recipes, like the ones found in this book, and working out together! Not only does this provide encouragement and a positive influence, it can help create a lasting bond.

Mothers are so often associated with food because that is who we depend on in our first years of life for food and nourishment. When we think about our comfort food as adults, so many times it goes back to what our mothers or grandmothers fed us as kids. Whether that food is lasagna or meatloaf, chances are we are comforted less by the actual food and more by the memories and feelings associated with it. For example, for me, one of my grandmothers cooked three hot meals a day. She didn't work outside the home and that is what she loved to do. She made the best breakfasts – homemade biscuits and jelly and eggs with runny yolks. To this day, eggs are still a favorite of mine and I eat them very often for dinner.

My mother was a single mom who worked multiple jobs. While we didn't have time for many sit-down meals, I can remember eating lots of bananas on the run. And my maternal grandmother also had a full-time job and I can remember peanut butter being a staple food for both her and my mother. As an adult, I eat a banana every day and peanut or almond butter several times a week. Lucky for me, these foods that I remember so well are not only healthful, but they are super affordable! As a mother, we all have the opportunity to influence our kids by being good role models. We often find ourselves doing things simply because our parents did. To ensure you leave a healthy impression on your kids, make sure they see you eat (and like) lots of vegetables, eat only one piece of (not the entire) cake, and spend more time being active than sitting on the couch or at the desk. Who says comfort food can't be vegetable lasagna made with whole grain pasta or turkey meatloaf?

Strong is the New Skinny

We all want the women in our lives to be around for a long time. In addition, we want them to stay strong as they age to help prevent falls, broken bones, and weak joints. Loss of bone density, osteoporosis, and osteoarthritis can be prevented through proper exercise.

Women need 180 minutes of exercise per week to protect themselves from bone-density loss, according to a study from the American Physiology Society. Plus, a study found that 16 weeks of resistance training increased bone density and elevated blood levels of bone density by 19%.

According to the Journal of Anatomy, *the strong muscles you develop while running can help protect against osteoarthritis. Also, the American Council on Exercise reports that strengthening and toning your lower body helps make your knees less vulnerable to injury. This is because stronger leg muscles have better control over your movements.*

I also encourage everyone to use Mother's Day as an opportunity to recognize the influence you are capable to have. Whether or not you have given birth to or are raising a child, you have the opportunity to influence everyone around you. The definition of mother as a verb is "to watch over, nourish, and protect" or "to bring up with care and affection". So, whether you're male or female, whether you've given birth or not, everyone is capable of "mothering". This Mother's Day, I encourage you to care for those you love by nourishing their bodies while also nourishing their souls. Each of us will leave our impact on this world and we each have a legacy to leave. Let's make sure it is a happy one and a healthful one! Obesity is 100% preventable and it starts by mothering.

My Don't Diet, Live It Meal for Mother's Day provides comfort and nourishment. Most every mother has made grilled cheese and tomato soup, and most every kid has enjoyed it! This is a family meal where comfort comes easy and healthful! Each dish is simple and soul-satisfying! The following recipes serve four.

Sweet Tomato Soup

<u>Ingredients</u>:
1 T extra virgin olive oil (EVOO)
½ cup diced onion
1 T chopped garlic
½ cup diced carrots
½ cup diced celery
½ t salt, ¼ t pepper
2 (14.5-ounce) cans no-salt-added diced tomatoes
3 roasted red peppers from a jar
16 ounces low sodium chicken or vegetable stock
<u>Directions</u>:
In a large Dutch oven, heat EVOO over medium-high heat. Add the onion, garlic, carrot, and celery and season with salt and pepper. Cook until the vegetables soften, about 10 minutes, then put them into a food processor with the diced tomatoes and roasted red peppers. Puree the mixture until smooth, then pour back into Dutch oven and stir in the stock. Simmer on low for 10 minutes.

You can serve immediately or refrigerate for up to one week. You can serve hot or chilled. A cold soup (like a Gazpacho) is great for summer months!

Roasted red peppers add a subtly sweet flavor to this tomato soup. Kids love the addition – as well as adults. Plus, red bell peppers contain more Vitamin C than oranges. They are also a good source of Vitamin A and beta-carotene. They are also one of the few foods that contain lycopene, which can prevent many known types of cancer! A satisfying and delicious life-preserver!

Gourmet Grilled Cheese

Ingredients:

2 T EVOO
8 slices whole grain bread
4 slices Monterey Jack, mozzarella, or provolone cheese
8 slices (approx. ½ lb) smoked deli turkey, chicken, or ham
2 handfuls of basil or spinach leaves
4 T grated parmesan or asiago cheese

Directions:

In a large skillet, heat EVOO over medium heat. If you can't fit four slices of bread in one skillet, prepare in two batches. While EVOO is heating, prepare sandwiches. Lay four slices of bread down and layer remaining ingredients (evenly distributed on each slice) in order, and top with last slice of bread. Add sandwiches to skillet. Cook for several minutes on each side, depending on brownness desired. Slice grilled sandwiches diagonally and serve with soup. They make great dunkers! Or, slice each sandwich into 4-6 mini squares and serve atop soup like glorious croutons!

This grilled cheese provides whole grains, calcium, protein, and lots of vitamins. Who knew a kid favorite could be so good for you! Now that feeds the body and soul!

Ginger Tea

Ingredients:
1 cup water
2-inch piece fresh ginger, peeled and thinly sliced (freeze remaining ginger for later use)
1 quart fresh brewed black or green tea, chilled
2 T agave syrup
Juice of 2 lemons or limes
1 cup sparkling water or club soda, chilled
Directions:
Prepare an hour ahead (up to 12 hours) by combining the water and ginger in a saucepan. Bring just to a boil, reduce the heat, and simmer about 5 minutes. Remove from heat and allow to cool. Strain ginger water and combine with remaining ingredients. Pour over ice in individual glasses.

Ginger has long been thought to have many health benefits, mainly alleviating nausea. Ginger can also act as an anti-inflammatory as well as aid in prevention of several types of cancer. An herbal remedy for whatever ails you – that's tasty comfort!

Chocolate Banana Boats

<u>Ingredients</u>:

4 ripe (but still firm) bananas

4 dark chocolate squares or 4 T dark chocolate chips (at least 70% cacao)

1 cup lowfat vanilla Greek yogurt or frozen yogurt

<u>Directions</u>:

Using a sharp knife, make a length-wise slit along the inner side of the unpeeled banana skin and almost through the banana. Push chocolate pieces into the slits and push banana skins closed. Wrap each banana tightly in aluminum foil. Place the banana packets in a 400-degree oven and cook for 10 minutes, flip halfway through cooking time. Allow to cool slightly. Open the banana packets and remove from foil. Serve on a plate and top with yogurt. Allow each person to scoop out their own banana boat and enjoy! Bananas have tryptophan – the same chemical that turkey contains. This mood regulating substance contains a level of protein that helps the mind relax so you feel happier. What a delightful way to end the meal and the day!

Chapter 6: June

Dad May Have Big Shoes to Fill, But Let's Keep His Belt Small

This month is Father's Day and a time for us to celebrate Dad. But as we celebrate, we should take time to think about the lifestyle Dad is living and how it might lead to fewer Father's Day celebrations. Does your dad currently struggle with his weight, fight blood pressure, and/or suffer from high cholesterol? Or maybe you are a man who is a dad, or wants to be a dad, who suffers from these heath woes yourself?

In many families, a "beer belly", "love handles", the "done-lap syndrome", etc. are used as jokes or punch lines about Dad and his physique. However, these are NOT terms of endearment and they should not be laughed at. When Dad, or anyone in the family, carries around extra weight it can lead to serious illness and disease such as coronary heart disease, type 2 diabetes, sleep apnea, gallbladder disease, osteoarthritis, colon and breast cancer, hypertension and stroke. I suggest we take Father's Day as a time to recognize the seriousness of being overweight or obese and do something about it.

Chances are your dad, or an influential man in your life, is overweight or obese – two out of three men are. So, you do have the power to make a difference. In fact, my dad has battled high triglycerides and high cholesterol for years. I am proud to say that he has his triglycerides under control and is greatly improved his cholesterol numbers. Not too long after I lost 50 pounds in college, my dad made some lifestyle changes and also lost some weight and in turn improved many of his health numbers. I am so proud of him – he's been my rock for so long, I want to make sure he sticks around!

A new study reports that life expectancy nationwide has increased by about four years for men and two years for women. However, the life expectancy has actually decreased for areas in the Deep South, Appalachia, and northern Texas. That's pretty bad and sad news for those of us here in the South. This University of Washington Seattle study indicates that obesity, high blood pressure, and tobacco use have all contributed to this decrease in life expectancy. All three of these factors can be reversed and are preventable ailments. It's been said that here in America, we are killing our kids through their food intake and their sedentary lifestyles. But, as it turns out, we adults are killing ourselves as well! We can't continue to eat the way we do and sit at desks, in cars, and on couches and expect to remain healthy.

Hard Work Pays Off

Father's Day is a perfect time for everyone to celebrate their dad and all the influential men in their life. They've supported us and cheered us on, and now it's our turn to return the favor. Let's remind the men in our lives that we want them to stick around for many more years. Being overweight or obese can take away what most father's consider to be their vital role – their ability to support the family. Obese men can expect to earn $7,000 less per year than a healthy-weight man. But, there is hope, by maintaining a healthy weight, fathers can enjoy a longer and more fruitful life.

Encourage dad to exercise so he can increase his office productivity. Exercising at least twice a week can help him feel more in control of his job. According to a survey in the International Journal of Workplace Health Management, *the benefits of workday workouts are as follows: Motivation improves by 32%, Time management improves by 28%, Concentration by 26%, Stress Management by 26%, Productivity by 25%, and Accuracy by 15%.*

I personally want to be able to celebrate many more Father's Days with my dad. He is a supportive man who has encouraged me and loved me more than he knows. And I am sure many of you have fathers who have done the same. So, use this Father's Day as the time to give back to Dad. Support him, encourage him, and love him enough to see him get healthy. Give Dad a pair of running shoes rather than a tie. Take Dad for a walk rather than a movie. Celebrate Dad with a healthful home-cooked meal rather than a greasy steak and loaded potato. He gave you his best for many years, now it's your turn to make sure Dad gets the best. Obesity is 100% preventable and it starts by celebrating Dad!

My Don't Diet, Live It Meal for Father's Day is my take on most every man's favorite meal – meat and potatoes! This meal is inspired by my dad and I know he loves these dishes. Your dad – or any man in your life – will love this meal as well. The following recipes serve eight. Leftovers are great the next day!

Dad's Meatloaf

Ingredients:
1 jar roasted red peppers – drained
2 T spicy brown mustard
2 T extra virgin olive oil (EVOO) + 1 T
½ cup diced onion
1 T chopped garlic
1 lb 93% lean ground beef, 1 lb 93% lean ground turkey
2 t Worcestershire sauce
1 cup egg substitute
¾ cup whole wheat bread crumbs (4-5 slices stale sandwich bread pulsed in food processor)
1 t salt, ½ t pepper

Directions:
Make sauce (up to a day ahead) by adding roasted peppers, mustard and 2 T EVOO to food processor. Pulse until smooth and creamy. Set aside (refrigerate if longer than 1 hour). Heat 1T EVOO in a large skillet on med-high heat, add onion and garlic. Cook until softened. Remove from heat and allow to cool. Once room temp, add to remaining ingredients along with ¼ cup of pepper sauce in large bowl. Mix gently with your hands. Transfer meat to a 9x13-inch baking dish (prepared with nonstick spray) and shape into a loaf about 5 inches wide and 3 inches high. Top with 1 cup of pepper sauce and bake for about 1 hour or until an instant-read thermometer registers 160 degrees. Allow to rest for 10 minutes before slicing. Serve with remaining pepper sauce as a drizzle over each slice.

This meatloaf is an excellent source of iron and protein. Beef keeps the flavor rich, while turkey cuts down on fat and calories. Don't tell anyone there is turkey in it and they'll never know! The roasted red pepper sauce is a huge hit with dads and kids alike. It's sweet, tangy, and much more flavorful than tomato sauce. Red peppers contain more vitamin C than an orange. This is not your typical meatloaf – it's much better tasting and way more healthful!

Smashed Potatoes

<u>Ingredients</u>:
3 lbs red potatoes, unpeeled, halved or quartered (depending on size)
1 T chopped garlic
1 T salt
½ cup lowfat buttermilk
½ cup skim milk
2 T butter
1 t salt, ½ t pepper
1 T fresh chives, scallions, or parsley (optional)
Few pinches of smoked paprika (optional)
<u>Directions</u>:
Place the potatoes, garlic, and 1 T salt in a large saucepan and cover with cold water. Bring to a boil, lower the heat, and simmer covered for 15-20 minutes. While potatoes are boiling, in a small saucepan, heat the buttermilk, milk, and butter over low heat. Once potatoes are fork tender, drain and return to warm pan. Smash with a potato masher then add ½ of milk mixture and salt and pepper. Continue smashing and adding warm milk mixture until you achieve desired consistency. Serve with fresh herbs or paprika.

Potatoes are a good source of vitamins C and B6, copper, potassium, manganese, and dietary fiber. Potatoes also contain a variety of phytonutrients that have antioxidant activity. Leaving skins on provides the biggest punch of all these nutrients. These tubers not only taste great, they are beneficial to your body!

Spiked Peach Tea

Ingredients:
2 quarts fresh brewed black tea – chilled
2 T agave syrup
2 fresh ripe peaches
8 ounces whiskey

Directions:
In a large pitcher, muddle (crush with end of wooden spoon) agave, 1 peach sliced, and ice. Pour chilled tea over mixture. To serve, pour tea into glass over ice. For dad and other adults add a shot of whiskey over ice before pouring tea. Serve with peach wedge for garnish. It's refreshing and delicious for kids, but also makes a manly drink for Dad – a healthful summer take on a man-favorite Long Island Iced Tea!

Peach Cobbler

Ingredients:
8 ripe peaches
Juice of 1 lemon
2 T agave syrup
¼ cup whole-wheat flour
¼ cup all-purpose flour
2 T plus 1 t sugar, divided
½ t baking powder
¼ t baking soda
¼ t salt
2 T chilled unsalted butter, cut into small pieces
1/3 cup lowfat buttermilk
2 T canola oil

Directions:
Heat oven to 400 degrees. Peel peaches and slice in wedges. Toss with lemon juice and agave. Add to 8x8-inch baking dish or 10-inch pie pan and cover with foil. Bake 15 minutes or until peaches are hot and juice bubbles. Remove from oven.

In a bowl whisk flours, 2 T sugar, baking powder, soda and salt. Cut in butter using two knives or pastry cutter until small pebble-sized pieces are formed. In a small bowl, whisk together buttermilk and oil and add to dry ingredients and mix until just moistened. Drop the batter onto fruit forming eight mounds. Sprinkle with the remaining sugar. Bake for 30 minutes, until fruit is bubbly and top is golden. Let stand for 10 minutes before serving.

Peaches are good sources of lycopene and lutein. These phytochemicals are especially beneficial in the prevention of heart disease, macular degeneration, and cancer. So, celebrate Father's Day with peach cobbler!

Chapter 7: July

Declare Your Independence this Fourth of July

This is the month America will celebrate its independence. It was July 4th, 1776 that America adopted the Declaration of Independence declaring its independence from Great Britain. While America as a country is no longer dependent, individual Americans and families have become grossly dependent on unhealthy food, technology, and comforts. These dependencies have led to a devastating obesity crisis which has led to further dependence on prescription medications to control blood sugar, cholesterol, and blood pressure. Today, the average American eats approximately 570 calories more EACH DAY than they did 30 years ago. To put that into perspective, those additional calories could lead to a weight gain of about a pound a week. That is 52 pounds a year!

What is so astonishing about this is that we can make a change. We do not have to risk our health and our future – obesity is widely reported as the #1 preventable cause of death in the United States. With two out of three adults and one out of three children overweight or obese, we are literally killing ourselves. The majority of Americans are affected by being overweight or obese. The main causes of this appear to be our dependence on supersize fast food meals, packaged "convenience" snack foods, sugary sodas and coffees, as well as our aversion to physical activity. We are eating more and moving less. Thirty years ago Americans were not only eating 570 fewer calories each day, they weren't sitting with an iPhone in one hand and a video game controller or remote control in the other. They entertained themselves by dancing in discos, playing in the cul-de-sac, roller-skating, playing Pac-Man while standing, and walking the streets with the ever-popular walkman.

Fitness for the Fourth

Fourth of July is a fun holiday that is typically spent at cookouts, hosting or attending parties, poolside, or lounging in the backyard. Here are ways you can burn some calories while also commemorating America's birthday:

- *Get ready for your cookout or party by mowing the lawn – use a push-mower and pull weeds by hand. You'll improve your appearance as well as your yard's!*

- *Swim with your kids, or swim alone. It can burn more than 500 calories an hour. Even if it's not proper (or pretty) form, just make sure you're not resting on the pool floor and you're moving both your arms and legs.*

- *Play tennis or badminton. Set up "court" in your backyard or even in the pool. You'll burn calories while having fun and developing teamwork among your family.*

- *Play old-school games with the entire family. Remember how much you used to enjoy Red Rover, Duck Duck Goose, Hide-&-Seek, Hopscotch, Leap Frog, and Three-Legged Race? They're enjoyable, engaging, and high energy.*

- *If you have enough people, play kickball, volleyball (even with a beach ball), baseball, touch football, or soccer. Everyone gets exercise and kids can develop eye-hand coordination as well as leadership skills!*

No matter what you do, don't just sit. Lawn chairs are uncomfortable and leave embarrassing marks on the backs your legs. So, get up, move, have fun, and celebrate our country!

Today, our entertainment typically involves us sitting down with fatty and/or sugary snacks on the couch or car seat next to us. We very rarely enjoy our meals at a table with a knife and fork. We want everything – information, dating, food, pleasure – instantly and single-handedly. Rather than eating a bowl of cereal and fruit, we eat a processed cereal bar, we send an electronic invitation to meet instead of walking over to ask in-person, we order food while sitting in a car only to consume it on the couch using our hands as utensils and laps as plates. American families rarely cook a healthful meal for the family, let the kids set the table, and sit down without the distraction of technology.

The good news? We can make a change today. Use Fourth of July as your day to declare your personal independence. We can sever our ties to processed foods and inactivity. We can make decisions that will help us lose our excess weight and gain our lives back. We can eat less and move more. We can declare our healthy independence and discover how much freedom we actually have – freedom from prescription medications, artery-clogging foods, and sedentariness. Obesity is 100% preventable – "We the People" can declare our independence!

My Don't Diet, Live It recipes for this month make for a fun, festive Fourth of July meal. It can be prepared on the backyard grill while your family waves sparklers or it can be made indoors while enjoying the AC before heading out to see professional fireworks. Either way, this scrumptious meal will provide fireworks in your mouth! It is perfect for kids and adults of all ages! The following recipes serve four.

Red White and Blue Sandwiches

<u>Ingredients</u>:

1 T extra virgin olive oil (EVOO)

½ cup lowfat plain Greek yogurt

1 T hot sauce (the heat will cook out for a nice flavor)

1 T chopped garlic

4 boneless skinless chicken breasts, 6 ounces apiece (use a meat mallet to pound down a larger breast and divide into two pieces if needed)

1 t salt, ½ t pepper

4 whole grain hamburger buns

4 T crumbled blue cheese (I recommend Gorgonzola)

Toppings: red leaf lettuce, sliced plum tomatoes, sliced roasted red peppers from a jar

<u>Directions</u>:

Combine first 5 ingredients in a large re-sealable bag. Add chicken to the bag and turn to coat chicken evenly. Allow to marinate in fridge for at least 8 hours, or overnight.

When ready to cook, remove chicken from bag and shake off excess marinade and season with salt and pepper. Grill for about 5-8 minutes on each side, depending on thickness of breast. Crumble 1 T of blue cheese on each breast and toast buns on grill during last 2 minutes. Serve "blue" chicken on buns with "red" toppings.

Blue cheese is an excellent option for topping your sandwiches and burgers – soft cheese typically have less fat and calories per serving because they have not had time to dry and become dense like hard cheese. Plus, blue cheese is full of flavor so you can use less while still getting the wonderful taste.

Watermelon Salad

<u>Ingredients</u>:
2 T white wine vinegar
Juice and zest of 1 lime
¼ cup EVOO
½ cup red onion, thinly sliced
4 cups seeded watermelon chunks
1 cup crumbled feta cheese
2 cups baby arugula
1 t salt, ½ t pepper

<u>Directions</u>:
Add the white wine vinegar, lime juice and zest to a small bowl. Whisk in the EVOO and season with salt and pepper. Add the thinly sliced red onion and let marinate for 5-10 minutes as you prepare the rest of the salad.

Add the watermelon, feta, and arugula to a large bowl. Toss with the vinaigrette and serve immediately after dressing.

This is a fun savory take on summer's staple melon! Again, we are using a soft cheese that is full of flavor. Arugula is a green with a tart, peppery flavor that pairs well with watermelon and feta. Arugula is an excellent source of vitamins A and C, folic acid, and calcium. Introducing these flavors to kids (and adults) helps develop their palates!

Red and Blue Brew

<u>Ingredients</u>:
16 ounces blueberry pomegranate juice
16 ounces soda water or seltzer water
4 ounces blueberry or lemon vodka (optional)
Blueberries and strawberries for garnish
Ice

<u>Directions</u>:
In a large pitcher, stir together first 2 ingredients. Serve in individual glasses with ice and add a shot of vodka if desired. Garnish with fresh berries.

Pomegranate juice is loaded with vitamins C and B5, potassium and polyphenol (an antioxidant found in red wine). The berries only add to the antioxidant content and the festive colors of Independence Day!

Patriotic Parfait

Ingredients:
4 slices store-bought angel food cake
1½ cups fresh blueberries
1½ cups fresh sliced strawberries
2 cups lowfat vanilla Greek yogurt OR light Cool Whip
Directions:
In individual tall glass dessert dish or cocktail glass, layer crumbled angel food cake, berries, and yogurt or whip in at least two layers. Use glasses tall enough to see the colorful layers. Garnish each glass with berries.

This is not only a festive Fourth of July dessert, it provides numerous nutrients. Blueberries are loaded with antioxidants and studies have shown they may improve memory! Both strawberries and blueberries are known to improve blood sugar levels and decrease risk of type 2 diabetes. This dessert looks fun, tastes great, and can make your future brighter!

Chapter 8: August

Growing Up and Feeling Down

Growing up is tough. I know from experience that being a kid and teen are some of the most challenging times in our lives. There are so many pressures associated with growing up – school, social life, puberty, changing bodies, media pressure, family issues, and countless more. I have been working with many kids and teens over the past few years teaching them to live healthfully before they reach adulthood. I can relate to these young people because I struggled with my weight growing up. I spent the majority of my adolescence embarrassed about the way I looked. I didn't look like the cheerleaders I went to school with and I didn't fit into the "cute" clothes girls my age were supposed to wear. My belly usually stuck out further than my chest. I can remember strategically tucking my shirt in the back so that it would blouse down in front and cover my stomach. I hated that my thighs rubbed together so badly when I walked that it created a rash. I had to think about which shorts to wear so they would not ride up between my thighs if I was going to walk in front of people.

These things I remember are still being experienced by kids and teens today. However, it is only amplified by the added pressure of instant gratification/abuse from social media. The kids I have worked with have struggled with health issues that run from anorexia to extreme overeating and complete inactivity to extreme exercising. However, they all suffer from the same cycle of comfort and self-hatred that result from being unhealthy. Many kids feel that they have no control over their life – parents' divorce, school work, sibling trouble, peer pressure – and it begins to manifest itself in the way we treat our bodies.

Part of the process of getting physically healthy is making a mind-body connection. In order to gain control of our health, we must be able to manage our thoughts and feelings about stress, food, our body, and life in general. That can be very hard, especially for a teenager.

Many kids find comfort in food. They become good at eating away and through emotions then sit around the house because they avoid social situations. This leads to a self-destructive cycle. Kids and teens need guidance, structure, and discipline. It may not be easy, but in order to find success, kids need to work hard.

Daily Assignment for Exercise

Are you feeling stressed, brain-dead, or losing sleep? Are your kids having trouble focusing on schoolwork or struggling with ADHD? You need a good dose of exercise! Yep, exercise can improve your brain as well as your body. Here are just a few ways it can help:

- *Exercise immediately elevates dopamine and norepinephrine (similar to Ritalin or Adderall). It controls impulses and allows the brain time to react.*

- *Exercise heightens senses and improves focus and mood. This eases tension and can lead to more motivation.*

- *Moderate exercise (30 minutes for adults, 20 minutes for children) results in a 5-10% improvement in cognition. The findings refer to executive function, the activity that takes place in the brain's frontal lobe.*

- *Regular exercise helps condition the body and mind for rest. A regular routine of physical activity can help you fall asleep faster and helps you get more out of the hours that you are asleep. So, you feel more rested, without getting more shut-eye when you exercise regularly.*

Luckily when I was growing up I played sports. There were times I was pushed outside my comfort zone, but that allowed me to progress and grow. It also gave me confidence that I could make changes and believe in myself. While change is never easy and no one likes leaving their comfort zone, some circumstances require it. And the best things in life are the ones that we work hardest for and fight for. Our health is definitely worth fighting for!

I know what it is like to grow up and feel down, but it does not have to be that way. Obesity is 100% preventable and it starts today!

My Don't Diet, Live It recipes for this month are geared toward getting back into the routine of school and extracurricular activities. It's a perfect time to start thinking about meals and snacks. Proper nutrition is vital this time of year because we need to feed our kids the proper fuel to keep their bodies and minds strong. These recipes are very affordable, which is great when you're buying notebooks, book bags, and clothes for back-to-school. Many of these can be prepared ahead of time and even with help from the kids! The lunches will stay safe even if left at room temp for a few hours. These are perfect lunches and snacks that even offer "extra credit"!

School Lunches

<u>Wraps and Pasta Salads</u>: Pair one of the wraps or pasta salads with one of the sides for a complete lunch. I love wraps and pasta because they are more durable and less likely to get soggy or smashed like sandwich bread can.

- Mexican Burrito: whole wheat tortilla stuffed with scrambled egg, veggies, cheese, and salsa. Extra Credit: This makes a great breakfast, lunch, or dinner. Plus, it can be served cold, hot, or room temp.
- The Elvis Wrap: whole wheat tortilla spread with 1 T peanut butter and topped with sliced banana. Extra Credit: This also makes a delicious breakfast and the beginning of an awesome dessert. Just drizzle with a bit of honey, fold over the wrap and put it on a grill or panini maker and you have an amazing dessert quesadilla.

- Italian Wrap: whole wheat tortilla stuffed with chicken, pesto, chopped grape tomatoes. Extra Credit: This offers a new flavor for kids in a familiar way. Chances are kids have enjoyed the same flavors in a pizza or tomato soup. If they're still unsure about pesto, just call it a pizza wrap.
- Asian Pasta Salad: whole grain pasta, brown rice, or quinoa, stir-fry veggie mix, sesame seeds, drizzled with low sodium soy sauce and extra virgin olive oil. Extra Credit: If you use the leftover veggies from your stir-fry the night before, you have a nearly no-cost lunch.
- Summer Pasta Salad: whole grain pasta, brown rice, or quinoa, sliced strawberries, crumbled goat cheese, chopped walnuts, drizzled with balsamic vinegar and extra virgin olive oil. Extra Credit: This utilizes affordable and sweet strawberries while they are still in-season while the cheese and nuts add in interesting flavor and texture that kids love.

Sides: Freeze the fruit or veggies the night before to help keep the rest of the lunch cold, and the produce will be perfectly crisp by lunchtime.
- 1 cup lowfat cottage cheese with frozen strawberries
- 1 string cheese, handful of baby carrots
- 1 cup lowfat Greek yogurt, handful of frozen red grapes
- 1 slice Swiss cheese wrapped around slices of bell pepper

After-School Snacks
These are extremely important so that kids are not literally running on empty. Most school lunches are at about 11 AM and without an after-school snack, kids would go 6-8 hours until dinner. We need to refuel every 4 hours.
- 1 handful of almonds, 1 peach or 1 cup broccoli
- Apple or banana with 1 tablespoon of peanut butter
- 1 cup of lowfat Greek yogurt with 1 cup blueberries
- Celery spread with 1 tablespoon of peanut butter and topped with raisins (ants on a log)
- Lean deli meat (turkey, roast beef) wrapped around slices of red or yellow bell pepper

49

- Coach D's Homemade Trail Mix: 1½ cups of whole unsalted walnuts (or almonds), 1½ cups of raisins (or cranberries or other dried fruit), 1½ cups of Cheerios (or Crispix, Wheat Chex, or Shredded Wheat), ¾ cup of dark chocolate chips (at least 60% cocoa). Combine all ingredients in large mixing bowl. Divide equally into seven individual ¾ cup portions and put into snack baggies. Extra Credit: This requires no refrigeration and is very resilient, which is great for an after-school snack. Since most kids don't go straight home after school, this can be stashed in a book bag, ball bag, instrument case, or purse and eaten at any time.

"Cool Crowd" Chocolate Milk

Ingredients:
4 T dark cocoa powder (I like Hershey's Special Dark)
4 t agave syrup
8 ounces warm water
32 ounces skim milk
Directions:
In a small bowl, combine first 3 ingredients, mix well. Add to cold milk in a large pitcher. Chill in fridge and serve cold. For an adult beverage, add a shot of vanilla vodka!
Dark cocoa powder is rich in flavonoids which are plant pigments that have antioxidant, anti-inflammatory, and antiviral properties. This is the same type of antioxidant found in green tea. The skim milk provides lots of calcium and Vitamin D. It's a healthy take on a childhood favorite!

While these recipes are geared towards kids, they are great for adults as well. And no matter your age or ability, you can make and enjoy these recipes! So, it's time to get back to school and back to health!

Chapter 9: September

Final "Fair" Days of Summer

During the month of September, especially in the South, we continue to enjoy the final days of summer – including state and county fairs and nights at the ballpark. I really enjoy these last moments of summer. However, there are still a few things we need to be wary of. Among these are a list of some frightful foods that can be found at cookouts, fairs, and ballparks. I encourage celebrating and enjoying all things in moderation. However, the following is a list of the foods we should avoid or limit whenever possible:

Deep-fried foods and snacks: You're at greater risk for high cholesterol and heart disease if you eat a diet that includes deep-fried or breaded foods, which are high in fat. Diets high in saturated fat and trans fats tend to raise cholesterol and blood pressure. When you fry foods that already contain saturated fat (like Twinkies at the fair), you simply add more fat to them. But even a fried veggie like the Bloomin' Onion has more than 800 calories, 58 grams of fat, 22 grams of saturated fat, plus 1,520 milligrams of sodium. These numbers don't include the dipping sauce, which is also loaded with fat, calories, and sodium.

Processed and refined carbs: Eating foods with fewer than three grams of fiber and more than ten grams of sugar (check the label to be sure) increases your risk for heart disease. Stick with whole wheat bread, whole grain cereals, and brown rice or whole grain pastas. If you're at a location that doesn't offer whole grain, enjoy an open-face sandwich (take off one piece of bread).

Hot dogs and bologna: Processed meats are fat and salt bombs, and they also contain nitrates, which have been linked to several types of cancer. Pick lean poultry or red meat, or even better, go for the seafood. Opt for grilled shrimp wrapped in a whole grain tortilla over a greasy chili dog.

<u>*Artificial sweeteners*</u>: Five hundred times as sweet as sugar and zero calories? Sounds pretty good, but studies show that those of us who use them are more likely to be overweight than not. The reason is that the sweet taste tricks your body to making you crave even more food, especially sweet stuff. Opt for natural sugars in fruit and veggies or add agave syrup to coffee or honey to your whole wheat toast. Limit diet sodas by choosing water with lemon or lime juice and sweetened with agave.

Fight Aging with Fitness

Each September, we celebrate National Grandparents' Day. Help your grandparents fight age-related ailments by getting them physically fit. And make sure you are a healthy grandparent by getting active today.

A study published in Medicine & Science in Sports & Exercise *found that strength training for an hour three times a week can help improve memory performance as you age. Plus, older adults' working memory performance increased by 14% after they strength trained three days a week for six months.*

Staying active cuts your risk of cognitive decline by about a third. And a 4,000-person study found that those who exercised had fewer symptoms of depression.

Risk of dementia later in life decreased by 26% for women who exercised at least once a week at age 30 versus those who didn't exercise at all.

Whether you're a granny or honoring grandpa, it's never too early or too late to fight aging by getting fit!

"Fortified" junk food: Don't be fooled by flashy nutritional claims on the front of a package – it's the label on the back you need to study. Avoid products that list sugar (or sucrose, fructose, etc) among the first three ingredients. And remember that "enriched flour" is just a fancy way of saying "refined white flour" – it has to be enriched because the refining process destroys most of the nutrients. Even kids' snacks like granola bars or "fruit snacks" can be loaded with sugar and not contain an ounce of real fruit. Choose real fruit and a handful of nuts over an energy bar or candy bar.

Enjoy the final days of summer – celebrate, relax, and spend time with your family and friends. Just make sure you also make smart choices to keep you healthy enough to enjoy many more in the future! Obesity is 100% preventable and we can start by savoring each moment...even these final "fair" days of summer.

My Don't Diet, Live It meal for September is a healthful one you can enjoy with your family in these final days of summer. Now is the time to get the very best out of the final days of the season. This meal uses the most flavorful seasonal ingredients, like peaches, arugula, and raspberries. The best seasonal meals are made of the tastiest ingredients and prepared in simple ways. It's delicious and nutritious. The following recipes serve four.

Grilled Pork and Peaches on Rocket
Ingredients:
4 thick-cut (1-inch) bone-in pork chops (8 ounces each)
4 firm peaches, halved and pitted
2 T extra virgin olive oil (EVOO)
1 t salt, ½ t pepper
4 cups arugula (aka rocket)
½ cup red onion, thinly sliced
¼ cup pine nuts
½ cup crumbled blue cheese
2 T balsamic vinegar plus 2 T EVOO, whisked together

<u>Directions</u>:
Preheat a grill on high. Brush pork chops and peach halves with EVOO. Season pork with salt and pepper. Grill pork for 4-5 minutes on each side. The outside should be slightly charred while still pink on the inside. Grill peaches flesh side down for about 5 minutes or until charred and softened. Note: if peaches are too ripe, they will turn to mush.

While pork and peaches grill, prepare rocket salad by tossing remaining ingredients in a bowl. Serve salad on a plate and top with a pork chop and sliced grilled peaches.

Pork compares favorably for fat, calories, and cholesterol with many other meats and poultry. In fact, cuts from the loin, like pork chops, are leaner than skinless chicken thighs. Plus, pork rivals milk as a source of riboflavin. Riboflavin plays an essential role in the release of energy from food, promotes growth and repair of tissues, and maintains healthy skin and eyes. Pick pork that is mostly pink (white spots are fat). Many times chops are fried, but pork can be a smart pick!

Arugula, also known as rocket, is slightly spicy and pairs perfectly with sweet peaches. It is a leafy green that stands out as a rich source of many vitamins and minerals. Compared with iceberg lettuce, arugula contains about eight times the calcium, five times the vitamin A, vitamin C and vitamin K, and four times the iron. Plus it also contains the antioxidants beta carotene and lutein which are known for the prevention of diseases like cancer and macular degeneration.

Pine nuts are nature's only source of pinoleic acid, which stimulates hormones and helps diminish appetite. Pine nuts also contain oleic acid which aids the liver in eliminating harmful triglycerides.

Raspberry Tea

<u>Ingredients</u>:
1 quart fresh brewed black or green tea – chilled
1 T agave syrup
¾ cup fresh raspberries, plus a few for garnish
Ice
<u>Directions</u>:
In individual glass or large pitcher, muddle (crush with end of wooden spoon) agave, raspberries, and ice. Pour chilled tea over mixture and serve with a few fresh raspberries on top! This tea is perfect any time of day. For a refreshing adult beverage, add a shot of whiskey or dark rum!
Tea contains healthful doses of antioxidants, or poylphenols that may ward off a range of diseases. Make sure to always brew your own – commercial bottled tea contains such small amounts of these antioxidants that you'd have to drink 20 bottles to get the polyphenols present in one cup of home-brewed tea. The fresh raspberries not only add sweetness, but even more nutrients and eye-appeal. Now that's invigorating!

Peach Melba Parfait

<u>Ingredients</u>:
2 cups fresh raspberries, plus a few for garnish
2 T agave syrup
2 ripe peaches, thinly sliced
4 cups lowfat vanilla Greek yogurt
<u>Directions</u>:
Combine raspberries and agave in a bowl. Mash with a large fork or potato masher until you get a chunky consistency similar to preserves.
In individual tall glass dessert dish or cocktail glass, layer yogurt, peaches, and mashed berries in at least two layers. Use glasses tall enough to see the colorful layers. Garnish each glass with a few raspberries or peach slice.
For this dessert, use peaches that are slightly riper than those in the pork dish since they aren't being cooked.

Chapter 10: October

Fall into a Healthful Season

As the weather gets cooler, we typically tend to stay inside more, eat heavier and richer foods, and sit on the couch watching football and all the new fall television shows. Also, the cooler weather allows us to hide any extra pounds with sweaters, jackets, and long pants. And this is only the beginning of a very extravagant few months starting with Halloween going into Thanksgiving and ending with Christmas and the New Year. But, we don't have to automatically give in to the abundance and allow our health to go by the wayside. If we focus on our personal health, we will start the next year without the regret and extra weight.

I encourage everyone to take advantage of the abundance of fantastic fall produce and gorgeous autumn weather. Here are some ways to get the benefit of this season and have a happy Halloween without the wicked weight gain:

- Some of the most nutrient-rich foods are in season during the fall months. Opt for squash (of any variety), sweet potatoes, cabbage, carrots, pears, apples, and plums. It's easy to eat for this season because all the colors that remind us of fall are the ones to eat now – bright orange, deep red, and rich green. Remember that the darker the vegetable or fruit – the higher the antioxidants and more vitamins it has. For you Hairspray fans or those who listened to Tupac in the '90's, then you know "the darker the berry, the sweeter the juice"! Since the produce is in season, it is cheaper and will taste better, so you don't need extra butter or sugar to make them taste good.

- Enjoy the fall weather as much as you can – the days are only getting shorter. So, take advantage of any daylight we have now before we lose that hour of daylight in the evenings when daylight savings time ends. Go out and take a walk to watch the sun set, rake leaves just to let your kids (or grandkids/nieces/nephews/neighbors) jump into the pile, walk through a pumpkin patch, winterize your house by cleaning up the yard, windows, basement, and attic. Getting rid of some of that clutter will burn calories – and reduce your fire hazards!

- Commit your extra hour to your health. While we miss the daylight in the evening, we will enjoy an extra hour when daylight savings time ends. So, make a commitment that you will dedicate that extra hour to doing something healthy – get in some extra physical activity, plan your family's fitness calendar for the entire month, plan and post your family's home-cooked meals for at least one week, go to a farmer's market and pick up fresh nutrient-rich produce, or cook a healthful meal with your loved ones.

- Watch eating too many empty calories around Halloween! I always buy candy that I don't like for the trick-or-treaters. That way I'm not tempted to eat what they don't. Also, if you happen to have candy in the house that you like, don't open the bag until the night of Halloween, or wait until the last minute to buy the candy.

- Allow yourself three or four pieces of candy on the night of Halloween. Spread out each piece so that you have a treat planned throughout the night. Some of your best bets if you do eat candy: twizzlers, tootsie rolls, junior mints, york peppermint patties, jolly ranchers, and dum dums. Remember that your teeth suffer just as much as your belly with too much candy. So spare your doctor and your dentist and limit your intake of the sugary treats. I suggest popping some popcorn and snacking on that throughout the evening rather than candy. Also try brushing your teeth or chewing a piece of sugar-free gum before the trick-or-treaters start arriving – the candy won't be as tempting with a minty fresh mouth.

Autumn is a beautiful season that brings many changes and opportunities. Don't let this be a season you fall into poor health habits – fall into a healthful routine that will keep you healthy this season and many more to come. Obesity is 100% preventable and it's the season to avoid wicked weight gain and fall into health!

Beat Breast Cancer

October is Breast Cancer Awareness month. Being overweight or obese increases the risk of breast cancer, as well as other health conditions and diseases including: Coronary heart disease, Type II diabetes, Sleep apnea, Gallbladder disease, Osteoarthritis, Colon cancer, Hypertension and Stroke. Reduce your risk of breast cancer by being active and staying at a healthy weight.

According to the National Cancer Institute, exercising four or more hours a week may decrease hormone levels and help lower breast cancer risk. More than two dozen studies have shown that women who exercise have a 30% to 40% lower risk of breast cancer than their sedentary peers.

Furthermore, one-third of breast cancer cases could be avoided through regular exercise and better nutrition, according to the International Agency for Research on Cancer. Plus, the more weight a woman gains from age 18 on, the more likely she is to have breast cancer later in life.

So, break a sweat, maintain a healthy weight, and spread the word to beat breast cancer!

My Don't Diet, Live It recipes for October are perfect for the night of Halloween as well as those Saturday and Sunday afternoons watching football. They are easy to whip up for the game day or Halloween night! Each dip and dipper can be mixed-and-matched. So, encourage guests to use their favorite dipper dunked in their favorite dip. Serve your favorite tea, wine, or champagne – make a "bar" and allow guests to garnish with orange-colored fruit for Halloween or any color that matches the team you're rooting for! The following recipes serve four, but can easily be doubled for a large game day or Halloween party.

Dipper #1: Pitas

Ingredients:
4 whole grain pitas
Olive oil flavor cooking spray
½ t garlic powder
½ t salt
Directions:
Preheat oven to 400 degrees. Put a large baking sheet in hot oven while preparing pitas. Cut pitas into triangles or strips. Remove pan and arrange pitas on hot pan without overlapping. Spray lightly with cooking spray and season with half garlic powder and salt. Bake at 400 for 3-4 minutes. Flip pitas over and lightly spray again with cooking spray and remaining garlic powder and salt. Bake for 3-4 minutes until pitas are crisp.

Dipper #2: Crudités

Ingredients:
Celery sticks
Carrot sticks
Cherry tomatoes
Cucumber slices
Yellow, orange, and red bell pepper strips
Cauliflower and broccoli florets

Directions:
Choose your favorite veggies –whether you prepare yourself or buy pre-cut in the produce section. Just aim for about 4 lbs of total veggies. Arrange on a large platter or set individual bowls filled with each veggie around the table. The more colorful, the better!

Dipper #3: Buffalo Chicken
Ingredients:
1 T extra virgin olive oil (EVOO)
2 T lowfat plain Greek yogurt
2 T hot sauce (Tabasco original or Chipotle flavor for less heat)
1 lb boneless skinless chicken tenders or fingers, cut into about 3 inch strips
Directions:
Preheat the broiler. In a large bowl, combine first three ingredients, add chicken and toss until the chicken is well coated. Allow to marinate up to 12 hours. Arrange the chicken on a baking sheet and broil 2-3 minutes. Flip chicken over and broil for additional 2-3 minutes. Serve with extra hot sauce.

Dip #1: Hummus
Ingredients:
1 (15-ounce) can chickpeas, rinsed and drained
2 roasted red peppers from a jar
¼ cup tahini (sesame paste, find in ethnic food section)
Juice of 1 lemon
2 T chopped garlic
1 t ground cumin
½ t salt, ¼ t pepper
3 T EVOO
Directions:
Place all ingredients (minus EVOO) in a food processor. Pulse to blend. Drizzle in EVOO until smooth and reaches desired consistency. Add a little water if needed. Transfer to a serving bowl or dish.

Dip #2: Roasted Garlic Dip

Ingredients:
1 head of garlic
1 t EVOO
½ cup lowfat sour cream
½ cup lowfat plain Greek yogurt
1-2 t Worcestershire sauce
½ t salt, ¼ t pepper

Directions:
Preheat oven to 400 degrees. Cut off top of head of garlic to expose the cloves, trimming about ¼-inch off top of each clove. Brush the cut cloves with EVOO then wrap in aluminum foil. Bake for 45 minutes. Remove, and allow to cool to room temp. Squeeze the garlic cloves out of their skins and into a mixing bowl. Mash well with a fork or whisk, then whisk in remaining ingredients. Refrigerate 2-4 hours to allow the flavors to meld.

Dip #3: Blue Cheese Dip

Ingredients:
1 cup lowfat plain Greek yogurt
1 T skim milk or lowfat buttermilk
1/3 cup crumbled blue cheese

Directions:
Whisk first 2 ingredients in a bowl. Add blue cheese, fold in to keep chunky or whisk to break up cheese crumbles. Refrigerate 2-4 hours to allow flavors to meld. Add an extra splash of skim milk or buttermilk to leftovers for a tasty salad dressing.

Chapter 11: November

Be Full of Thanks Not Food and Frenzy

With Thanksgiving right around the corner, it's the time of year when we all seem to be filled with stress, to-do lists, anxiety, the turkey dinner, and other holiday foods. Thanksgiving is the beginning of a two-month period where most of us put the festivities ahead of our health. The holidays can be a very hard time to stay healthy and maintain your weight, much less lose weight. Several studies have shown that the average American gains anywhere from three to 12 pounds during the period from Thanksgiving to New Year. So, I encourage everyone to kick-off this season by being full of thanks this Thanksgiving and taking the focus off of the food and frenzy. Here is my plan to tackle Turkey Day and get a healthful head start to the holidays:

Eat Breakfast: On Thanksgiving morning, wake up and eat a healthy and hearty breakfast. Go for a mix of protein and carbs like peanut butter on toast with an apple or pear; an egg with a slice of cheese on a whole wheat English muffin with a bowl of raspberries or blueberries; or a bowl of oatmeal made with skim milk and a banana.

Water: Drink lots of water throughout the day. About 30 minutes before you are scheduled to eat, drink a glass of water. Avoid sodas, sweet teas, and any pre-made drinks. These are loaded with sugar. If you're unsure, red wine is always a good choice. If you have more than a few alcoholic drinks, alternate a glass of water between each drink.

Appetizers/Snacks: Avoid the urge to eat mindlessly. If trays of food are put in front of you, don't grab for things just because they are there. Avoid creamy dips with buttery crackers. Stick with veggie platters or baked tortillas or pita chips with salsa or hummus. A handful of nuts are better than greasy chips or crackers. Also, wait as long as possible before you give in to the first bite of the appetizer. Once you start, it's hard to stop. So, chew a piece of gum or pop a mint to keep your mouth fresh.

Turkey: Turkey is a better choice than ham. Dark meat turkey does have more fat than white meat, but it also contains more iron and zinc than white meat. Plus, it has more flavor and doesn't dry out as easily, so you may need to pour on less gravy. Or, better yet, pick cranberry sauce which is a healthier condiment than gravy. Whether you pick white or dark, you should always remove the skin because that is where the truly unhealthy fats are found.

Sides: Make your plate as colorful as possible. Try to limit mashed potatoes and gravy and go for sweet potatoes. For my meal, I add a bit of real maple syrup to mashed potatoes and I replace marshmallows with a walnut topping. If making your own isn't an option, you can remove the marshmallow topping to save calories. Green vegetables can be good, although at this time of year, they can be loaded with cream and fat in a casserole. Instead of creamy green beans topped with fried onions, I toss my green beans with sliced almonds. Avoid creamy-looking casseroles and dishes with "crumble" toppings. These are typically just greasy crackers with added butter.

Bread: Avoid adding rolls or muffins to your plate. You will get plenty of starch from everything else on the menu like potatoes and stuffing. If you must have bread, go for just one piece and don't add butter.

Dessert: Stick to pumpkin or sweet potato pies. Both of these are healthier than pecan or apple. Avoid any pies with a double crust. Crust is very fattening because the main ingredient is shortening, butter, or lard. If you must have two slices of pie, eat only the filling, don't eat the end crust. You'll save calories and still get the best part. Also, try to avoid adding whipped cream or ice cream and just enjoy the taste of the dessert. Eat it slowly and enjoy it.

Stick to your Faves: Don't put something on your plate if you aren't that excited about eating it. Save the calories for something you'll enjoy. Furthermore, if you put something on your plate thinking you will like it but don't, you do NOT have to eat it just because it's on your plate. Even if old Aunt Mable thinks you should eat more, just smile and tell the old lady how wonderful everything was.

<u>*Second Helpings*</u>: Don't immediately go back for seconds. It takes 20 minutes for our brains to register that our stomachs are full. So, if you hoover through two plates of food, you will likely have overeaten which will lead to feeling severely uncomfortable for the rest of the day.

<u>*Get Moving*</u>: While watching the traditional Thanksgiving Day football game, don't sit for any period longer than an hour. Get up during a commercial break and walk around. After you eat, take a walk around the block, or take your kids out for a game of football or tag. Or, impress your family and take out the trash, walk the dog, help clean up the dishes, or start putting up Christmas lights and decorations!

With these tips and ideas for the holidays, you and your family will fill up on thanks rather than the food and frenzy of the season. Let's be thankful that obesity is 100% preventable and make a change today!

Sweat to Stop Smoking

The American Cancer Society marks the Great American Smokeout every year in November to encourage smokers to quit. You can increase your chances of quitting for good by exercising.

Ex-smokers who start exercising after they quit are more likely to stay smoke-free, reports a study in the journal Preventive Medicine. *Those who increased their activity by 16% were 84% more likely to be smoke-free than those who exercised less. Exercise reinforces your commitment to a healthy lifestyle and can help battle withdrawal-related fatigue and sleep problems.*

Further, working out may stop your urge to smoke. Women in an eight-week smoking cessation program received patches and counseling, but those who also walked briskly for 50 minutes three times a week reported fewer cravings. So, workout to smokeout!

My Don't Diet, Live It recipes for November are my personal recipes that I make every year. They are all side dishes and a beverage that are fantastic for Thanksgiving Day, whether you are hosting or taking a dish. They are easy and healthful, and much of the work can be done ahead of time. The following recipes serve eight.

Sweet Potato Casserole

Ingredients:
4 lbs sweet potatoes
2-4 T real maple syrup (not flavored pancake syrup)
1 T butter
1 t vanilla
1 t cinnamon
¼ t each nutmeg and ginger
Ingredients for crumble topping:
½ cup chopped walnuts (or almonds or pecans)
2 T brown sugar
1 T flour (I use whole wheat flour)
½ t cinnamon
1 T cold butter
Directions:
Bake whole sweet potatoes (with skin on) at 400 degrees until tender (30-60 minutes depending on thickness of potatoes). Allow to cool, then peel and add to a large bowl. Add other ingredients and beat with potato masher or hand mixer. In a separate bowl, combine ingredients for crumble topping and mix well with fingers. Pour sweet potatoes into a casserole dish or pie/cake pan. Sprinkle crumble topping over the top. You can make ahead up until this point and keep in fridge overnight or at room temp for up to an hour. To serve, bake at 350 degrees for 15-30 minutes, or until nuts are browned and crumble topping is set.

Sweet potatoes contain a wealth of orange-hued carotenoid pigments, including vitamin A and beta-carotene. In fact, sweet potatoes can be a better source of beta-carotene than green leafy vegetables. They are also standouts for providing a number of antioxidant and anti-inflammatory nutrients. Now that's sweet!

Green Beans

<u>Ingredients</u>:
2 lbs frozen green beans
4 ounces pancetta (or bacon), thick-sliced
½ t salt, ¼ t pepper
¼ cup sliced almonds
<u>Directions</u>:
Steam green beans in a microwave-safe container with about ¼ cup water. Heat on high for 4-5 minute increments until beans are softened, but still very crisp. Remove and immediately drain and allow to cool. Meanwhile, dice pancetta into ¼-inch pieces and add to a large sauté pan. Turn on medium heat and render the pancetta until just crisp. Remove pancetta from pan, leaving the grease in pan. Add the green beans to the warm pan and cook in the pancetta drippings just to warm beans. Transfer the beans to the serving bowl. Taste one bean to see if salt and pepper is needed. Since pancetta is salty and peppery, you may not need it. Top green beans with crispy pancetta and sliced almonds. Serve immediately.

Green beans are an excellent source of Vitamin K and other antioxidants, even better than green peas. Vitamin K is fat-soluble, so adding a little pancetta and almonds will only boost your body's absorption of nutrients in this delish dish!

Cranberry Relish

<u>Ingredients</u>:
2 12-ounce bags fresh cranberries (if not in-season, use frozen)
¼ cup dried cranberries
Zest and juice of 1 large grapefruit
2 T spicy brown mustard
1 t salt
1 cup water, plus more if needed
<u>Directions</u>:
Add all ingredients to a large pot and heat on medium-high. Stir really well to ensure it does not stick to bottom of pan. As the cranberries cook, they will begin to burst. Once they begin to burst, turn heat down to low and allow to cook for about 5 minutes, stirring occasionally. Remove from heat. I like to have a mix of whole and mashed cranberries, but if you prefer a smoother relish, mash with a fork or potato masher. You may also wish to add more water as the relish cools depending on your desired consistency. You can serve warm or make ahead and serve cold or room temp.

This is a much fresher, less sweet, and much more flavorful alternative to the canned cranberry sauce. Trust me, your guests will love this version. It is great as a spread, dip, and even by the spoonful! I make this year-round and use it as a spread on chicken or turkey sandwiches. It keeps in the fridge for about a month and freezes for at least 6 months. Buy extra bags of fresh cranberries while they are in-season and throw them in the freezer (in the bag they come in) to have all year long.

The phytonutrients in cranberries have long been known for protection again urinary tract infections. This is because those nutrients are anti-bacterial and can actually ward off infections in your mouth, gums, and stomach as well. That makes for a relish to relish!

Apple Cider Cocktail

<u>Ingredients</u>:

32 ounces no-sugar-added apple cider

8 ounces whiskey OR ½ cup water + 1 T apple cider vinegar + 1 T vanilla extract

8 cinnamon sticks and 8 slices apple for garnish (optional)

<u>Directions</u>:

This drink can be served ice cold or warm. My guests love it ice cold, so I keep the cider in the fridge and whiskey in the freezer. I add 4 ounces cider and 1 ounces whiskey (or ½ ounces apple cider/vanilla mixture) to a cocktail glass and garnish with a cinnamon stick and apple slice. If your guests want a warm cider, heat the cider over low heat (should be just under a simmer) and add room temp whiskey (or apple cider/vanilla mixture) as you serve and garnish.

This is a delicious seasonal beverage that satisfies all ages without all the added sugar or fat of typical holiday drinks.

Chapter 12: December

Break from Holiday Stressing to Savor Life's Blessings

This is the time of year when the hustle and bustle of the season can take over our lives. The consumer appeal of the mall and online shopping overshadow the blessings that take place right before our very eyes. These daily blessings are even more evident during the holidays – all we have to do is open our eyes and truly see what really matters.

Luckily for me, over the past few years my family and close friends have agreed to forgo material gifts for the gift of time together. We celebrate the holiday with festive and delicious food, cheerful beverages, fun games, and spending quality time together. Let's face it, this time next year when you look back on the holiday season, will you be able to remember each present that you received and from whom you received it? Or will you remember the conversations, experiences, and love you shared?

As I look back on the Christmases from my childhood through today, what comes to mind are the shared memories, traditions – new and old, laughs, and love. Growing up, our Christmas season started with the annual trip to our farm to cut down our tree. My dad and I would put on old jeans, good "work" shoes, and hefty gloves and take a ride out to the farm. We started looking and would pick out ones we thought were contenders as we made our way through the woods. We always chose three – one big one for Mom's house, a medium one for Dad's house, and a small one for Granny's house.

Unfortunately, many of the loved ones with whom I shared Christmas experiences have now left this earth, but will never leave my heart. Some of my favorite Christmas memories involve my Granmommie and Granny.

One of my favorite memories is our annual drive up to Kentucky to see my Granmommie. We would typically arrive late in the evening and my mom and I always bet on whether Granmommie fell asleep while waiting for us. Once we arrived, Granmommie had homemade Chex mix, "soup beans", and banana bread waiting for us. I adored being able to fall asleep next to Granmommie under an extra blanket she always added just for me.

I can also remember going to Granny's house for Christmas dinner – complete with dressing in a cast-iron skillet and the best chess pie I've ever had. The next morning started with homemade biscuits in that same skillet topped with homemade plum jelly. I loved opening presents at Granny's because I knew each year one of my gifts would be a year-long experience. My dad got me a season pass to Opryland every year (any native Middle Tennessean from the 1980's or 1990's will understand that). He usually wrapped it in a large box with a pack of size-D batteries or multiple boxes inside each other. I loved that he made opening the gift an experience.

I cherish those memories. They are sights, sounds, smells, and love that can never be replaced. I do not remember details of exactly what I got (or didn't get) for Christmas – I don't remember the specifics of what was under the tree, but rather what happened around it each year. Are the tasks that top your to-do list things that your loved ones will truly cherish? If not, maybe it's time to take a step back from the holiday stress and appreciate your true blessings.

I became a health and weight loss coach because I want people to make memories for as many years as they can. My goal for clients is not an ideal weight, but rather to give them a better life. You don't have to be a size 2 or at your high school weight to be healthy. You can make small changes now to help you get and stay healthy so you can continue to make memories with your loved ones for many Christmases to come.

I wish I could have my grandparents here to celebrate Christmas every year. While I can't have that, I can take care of myself and help keep my loved ones healthy so we can love and laugh through future holidays and cherish past holidays.

Save Time to Savor the Season

During the holidays, no one has any time to waste. Luckily, working out doesn't have to take forever. Going hard for just 20-30 minutes can actually provide more benefits than exercising at a moderate pace for twice as long.

For example, people who cycled at a high intensity for 20 minutes torched more calories for hours after their workouts than they did after cycling at a low intensity for 30-60 minutes, according to a study reported in Medicine & Science in Sports & Exercise.

Brief workouts with heavy weights may be best for blasting fat, according to an Italian study. One group did 32 minutes of interval-style lifting with heavy weights while another group did 62 minutes of lighter lifts with more reps. Over the next 22 hours, the heavy lifters burned an extra 363 calories. Your muscles work harder with interval training (periods of intense exertion alternating with periods of lighter exertion or rest), so they have to do more post-workout rebuilding. That burns calories and lifts metabolism-boosting hormones.

A Colorado State University study found that people burn an additional 242 calories in a day when they performed 25 minutes of interval training.

A study published in the International Journal of Obesity *revealed that women who did 20 minutes of interval training three days a week lost an average of 5.5 pounds over 15 weeks. Meanwhile, women who performed 40 minutes of steady-state aerobic exercise three days a week gained about a pound during the same period.*

If thoughts of gift shopping and wrapping, party planning, and holiday decorating have you stressing, it's time to take a break and count your blessings. Make memories that last a lifetime, and do what you can to make sure you are here to make future memories. Obesity is 100% preventable and that is definitely a blessing!

My Don't Diet, Live It recipes for December are fantastic and festive dishes that are perfect for any holiday party. You can make and serve them all together at your party, or add one to your holiday menu or take one to a party you are attending. They will be enjoyed all season long! The serving sizes are noted on each of the following recipes.

Holiday Potato Skins

Ingredients:
16 medium sized red potatoes (about 3 lbs total)
1 T extra virgin olive oil (EVOO)
1 T chopped garlic
½ cup diced onion
½ cup frozen peas
½ cup lowfat plain Greek yogurt (or lowfat sour cream or Neufchatel cheese)
1 T butter
½ t salt, ¼ t pepper
1 roasted red pepper from a jar, sliced into 16 1-inch strips
Directions:
Add potatoes to a large pot of water and bring to a boil. Boil for about 4 minutes. Check with a fork to see if they have softened. You want them to still be fairly firm (because they need to hold their shape and they will be baked again). Remove from heat, drain potatoes and allow to cool and dry.
Meanwhile, heat EVOO in a sauté pan over medium low heat and add garlic and onion. Sauté for 5-10 minutes, stirring regularly, until onions have browned slightly. Turn off heat and add peas. Allow this mixture to cool.

Once potatoes are cool, slice in half and scoop out some of the flesh, leaving about ¼-inch of the flesh with the potato skin. Add scooped out potato, plus onion and pea mixture, yogurt, butter, salt, and pepper, to a food processor. Pulse until mixture is combined and smooth, but not whipped. It should be a light green color.

Fill each of the potato skin with the mixture. Place each skin on a baking sheet and bake at 350 degrees for 10-15 minutes. Watch closely for browning of the edge of the skins, you want them to be golden brown and the filling to be warmed through. Remove from oven and place on a serving platter. Top each skin with a roasted red pepper strip to serve.

These are perfect for a party because they are an adorable holiday-colored finger food. They are great hot, but they can sit out and be enjoyed at room temp. Plus, red potatoes are high in iron, vitamin C, potassium, and fiber. Your guests will love this potato skin, and they won't even miss the bacon, cheese, and high-fat sour cream!

Makes about 4 dinner or 8 cocktail party servings.

Salmon Cakes

Ingredients:

4 (5-ounce) canned or pouched salmon, drained well

1 cup whole wheat bread crumbs (4-5 slices stale sandwich bread pulsed in food processor)

1 cup egg substitute

2 rounded teaspoons Old Bay seasoning blend

2 roasted red peppers from a jar, finely diced

1 t hot sauce

2 to 3 T fresh dill and/or chives, finely chopped

Juice and zest of 1 lemon, plus 1 lemon for garnish

½ t salt, ¼ t pepper

2 T extra virgin olive oil (EVOO)

½ cup lowfat plain Greek yogurt (or or Neufchatel cheese)

½ cup chili sauce (not cocktail sauce which is loaded with sugar)

Directions:

Combine the first 9 ingredients in a large bowl, using clean hands. Separate into 4 equal portions and make 2 cakes or patties out of each portion (total of 8 cakes). If making for a cocktail party, you can make them more bite-size and split each patty again making a total of 16 cakes. In a large nonstick sauté pan, heat 1 T of EVOO over med-high heat and add half of the cakes. Cook for 3 minutes, then flip and cook another 3 minutes. Remove cakes to a baking sheet fitted with a rack and put in a low (250-degree) oven to keep warm. Add the remaining 1 T of EVOO to the same pan and cook remaining cakes. Add last cakes to warm oven.

In a small bowl, whisk together yogurt and chili sauce. Serve cakes with dollop of sauce and a lemon wedge.

This is a super healthy and tasty take on crab cakes. They are great for dinner, and perfect for a holiday cocktail party. Salmon provides a wallop of omega-3's and heart-healthy fats. Canned or pouched salmon has a less fishy taste than fresh, so it is perfect even for kids (or adults) who say they don't like fish!

Makes about 4 dinner or 8 cocktail party servings.

Bread Pudding Bundles

Ingredients:

8 whole wheat hot dog or hamburger buns (buy when they are on sale and keep in freezer)

1½ cups egg substitute (you can use 4 eggs if you want it richer)

2 cups skim or lowfat milk

1 T vanilla (or whiskey)

1 t cinnamon

¼ cup brown sugar

¼ cup maple syrup

2 T melted butter

Optional add-ins: ½ cup of your choice of chopped walnuts, chopped pecans, raisins, dark chocolate chips, candied ginger, or diced apple

Maple syrup for drizzling

Directions:
This recipe works great with frozen bread. I pull out a package of whole wheat buns that I bought on sale and have kept in the freezer (up to 6 months). Break or cut up the buns into bite-size pieces and lay in one layer on a baking sheet. Bake at 250 degrees for about 15-30 minutes, flipping bread occasionally. You want the bread to dry out, but not get crispy. Remove from heat and allow to cool.

Meanwhile, whisk remaining ingredients in a large bowl. Add cooled bread and mix well. Allow to soak for at least 2 hours, even better overnight. Just cover and keep in fridge. Once you are ready to bake, remove bread mixture from fridge and add optional add-ins (you can also leave plain). Prepare a muffin tin with cooking spray. Scoop bread pudding mixture into muffin tin. To ensure bread pudding stays moist, I prefer to bake in a water bath (you don't have to do this, and can skip this if you are in a hurry or like a crispier bread pudding). Place muffin tin in a large baking/roasting pan with sides that come up to the top of the muffin pan. Fill the large pan with water so that the water comes to halfway up the muffin cups. Carefully place the water bath in the oven (preheated to 350 degrees) and bake for about 20-30 minutes. Check occasionally for doneness – it should spring back on the top and a toothpick should come out clean. Don't over bake or allow the edges to get too brown. Remove from oven and allow to cool for 5 minutes, then immediately remove bread pudding bundles from pan. Serve with a drizzle of warm maple syrup.

This whole wheat version of bread pudding is a favorite of mine. It is not as rich or sweet as traditional bread pudding and is more like a moist baked French toast. It is perfect for the holidays because it works for holiday brunches, cocktail parties, or as a dessert for dinner. It is perfect any time of day and can be prepared ahead of time and baked at the last minute.

Makes 8-12 servings.

Cranberry Bellini

Ingredients:

16 ounces no-sugar-added 100% cranberry juice (not juice cocktail)

16 ounces champagne, Prosecco, or sparkling cider

4 ounces Grand Marnier or orange liqueur (optional)

8 slices orange for garnish (optional)

Directions:

This drink can be prepared ahead of time in a large pitcher, but the sparkling wine/cider will lose the fizz after a couple hours. So I prepare my glasses individually, keeping all the ingredients in the fridge. I add 4 ounces each of the cranberry juice and sparkling wine/cider and ½ ounces Grand Marnier to a cocktail glass and garnish with an orange slice.

This makes a delicious festive beverage for cocktail parties or holiday events. You can even serve one version for adults and one for kids and those who don't drink alcohol. Just use different glasses for cocktails and mocktails.

Makes 8 servings.